A Woman's Story

Following the Light through
Addiction, Trauma and Abuse

Darlene A Hill

A Woman's Story
Copyright © 2021 by Darlene A Hill

All rights reserved. No part of this publication may be reproduced, distributed, or transmitted in any form or by any means, including photocopying, recording, or other electronic or mechanical methods, without the prior written permission of the author, except in the case of brief quotations embodied in critical reviews and certain other non-commercial uses permitted by copyright law.

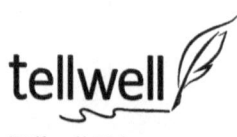

Tellwell Talent
www.tellwell.ca

ISBN
978-0-2288-5205-6 (Paperback)
978-0-2288-5206-3 (eBook)

A BOOK ABOUT ME…

LOVINGLY DEDICATED TO MY DAUGHTERS;
CHRISTINE, LISA AND ELISABETH

A woman's story is about growing up with a narcissist mother and a WW11 Vet father; a story about abuse, pain and mental health problems; including PTSD, depression, anxiety, broken marriages and compulsive gambling, while raising three daughters and falling in a "forever" love.

TABLE OF CONTENTS

Chapter 1 GROWING UP 1
Chapter 2 ABUSE AND BROKEN MARRIAGES 8
Chapter 3 BACK TO SCHOOL (AGAIN) 23
Chapter 4 SOUL MATES 26
Chapter 5 RAISING TEENAGE DAUGHTERS 45
Chapter 6 MY MENTAL HEALTH 49
Chapter 7 LOSS 57
Chapter 8 RECOVERY AND HOPE 62

AUTHORS NOTE 68
ACKNOWLEDGEMENTS 70
LIST OF HELPFUL RESOURCES 71

WITH LOVE AND APPRECIATION

Chapter 8 never would have happened the way it did without the loving support of my family; especially true of my husband **Rob**, my brothers **Bill** and **Bob** and my sister-in law **Mona**. To each of you, I thank you.

A WOMAN'S STORY 2020/2021
BY DARLENE ANNE HILL
Port Alberni, B.C. Canada

CHAPTER 1

GROWING UP

We grew up poor and we grew up fast my four brothers and me. Mom was a narcissist through and through. She was manipulative and mean and yet if you were to ask her, she was always the victim...

Dad, on the other hand was a WW11 survivor. He was strict. Corporal punishment was doled out swiftly. He never said "I love you" yet somehow, we all knew he did love us. In his own way of course. We grew up with the old adage that "children should be seen and not heard" and we should "only speak when spoken to."

My four brothers are actually "half" brothers as my mom was married before she met my dad. I also have five other half siblings from my dad's side; I remember meeting them, but I don't know them. My four brothers, Nick, Don, Bob and Bill are, as far as we're concerned, true siblings. My dad, for the most part, raised them and therefore all of us kids referred to him as dad.

My oldest brother, Nick, is 18 years older than me and he took on a more parental role with me and our other siblings. Our mom wasn't around a lot and that left a lot of the adult responsibility to Nick. Understandably, Nick resented this and as a result we didn't get along very well in my formative years. My second oldest brother, Don, who is 14 years my senior and I are not close and although our relationship is estranged, when we do get together, we appear close and are kind to one another. Next in the lineage comes my brother Bob. He is 11 years older than me. Bob is awesome; he is gentle, kind and caring and that's how I remember him growing up and how he remains to be today. I love my big brother Bob and trust in him wholeheartedly.

I was born in Burnaby, B.C. and we moved to Vancouver Island when I was five years old. We moved around a lot, usually every two years; either the house was too big or too small or my parents didn't like the location.

As a result, I attended almost every school in our community of Port Alberni, B.C. The advantages to that were that I got to meet a lot of good people and fortunately I made friends easily. Although I wasn't allowed friends over to my house, I was from the era that children spent all our free time outside only coming in at the end of each day when the street lights came on. Childhood was fun with friends; we played a lot of games and rode our bikes for hours.

When I was about seven or eight years-old I started going to church. My parents didn't go, but I started going with a friend from school so that I could join Brownies. I was in Brownies then Girl Guides and then Messengers. My mom was not supportive, I had to argue to go and promise to use my allowance for expenses and weekly dues. In reference to attending Messengers, my mom was really jealous of my leader; she would cry and complain about me spending so much time with her; stating that it "wasn't right" for "THAT woman to be spending time with other people's daughters." For me I enjoyed meeting once a week and doing crafts, I remember we all sat around a big table and drank tea, made crafts and laughed a lot. I felt warm and cared for, but the guilt that my mom placed upon me was too much to bear, so I quit going to appease her.

My parents were not a loving family and I don't recall either of them showing us any affection. Other than one time when I got a cold, I remember my mom rubbing a cold medicine on my chest and back. Otherwise, we were pretty much left on our own. I'd come home from school by myself and wouldn't see anyone until dinner time usually around 6:00. I remember only being allowed to bath once a week and that was using my mom's left-over bath water. (She'd bathe almost every night). I remember crying because I'd have to go to school with greasy hair and my mom saying "too bad." She used to cut my hair to, and believe me when I say she couldn't (or wouldn't) cut my hair nicely. Looking back, I'm surprised I made friends so easily.

I also remember the only time my dad would hold me was if I fell asleep in the car then he'd carry me in the house and put me to bed. I used to fake fall asleep in the car as often as I could get away with it.

My childhood summers were spent with my brothers Nick and Bob and their families, because they were so much older than I was, they were already married and had children of their own. It wasn't until late in my adulthood that I learned from Nick that mom would simply drop me off at his place at the beginning of summer and would pick me up in time for the new school year. I can recall driving the 500 miles to my brothers places in Prince George each summer, I always thought that I had been invited, but unbeknownst to me I had been "dumped" on my brother's doorstep. Despite this I have mostly good memories of being at my brothers, especially true of Bob and Mona. Their home was filled with love and laughter, whereas Nick's home was filled with anger, resentment and a lot of hostility. I used to beg my mom not to make me go to Nick's, but she said that I had to go. When at Bob and Mona's my summers were filled with drive-in movies, lake fishing and swimming at the river. As I got older, I would babysit my nieces and nephews too.

Nick's wife, Marita would talk to me from time to time and ask me why I didn't like to stay at their place, I do not recall what my response was, I don't know if I told her that I was scared of them, I likely just shrugged my shoulders and said "I don't know." I do recall, however, how scared I was when I stayed with them. They were very strict and they physically punished their two daughters whenever they felt the need. Their third child, a little boy, was rarely, if ever punished, at least when I was around. I do remember one time when the girls were being disciplined, I took my little nephew and we hid in the closet until the punishment had been doled out. I know he cried and I tried my best to console him through my own tears.

I recall one Sunday afternoon when I was about 10 years old or so, my mom took me aside and her and my dad's sister, my auntie Margery, told me I was getting fat (I wasn't ever overweight as a child) and that no man would ever want to marry a fat girl. I recall being reduced to tears, my mom said it was for my own good and that I needed to hear it. I've never forgotten how this made me feel as a young child; inadequate and ashamed.

At the age of 55 my dad was diagnosed with early onset Alzheimer's Disease; I was 11 years old. He died shortly after my 21st Birthday, after languishing in a Veteran's hospital for seven years. Alzheimer's Disease was not well understood then, sadly my dad thought it was God's way of punishing him for not being more understanding of people with special needs. All we understood about the disease was that it was slowly killing my dad's brain. He also thought if he tried hard enough, he could retrain his brain. He sought out my help and at the age of 12, I remember trying to teach my dad the alphabet. We would sit on the edge of his bed and I would print out the alphabet, he would try and memorize it and then he'd trace over my letters trying to relearn how to print again. This memory causes me sadness, because I remember how hard my dad struggled to learn. Again, I felt inadequate, because I wasn't able to help my dad.

When learning the alphabet didn't work, my dad asked me several times to help him commit suicide. He apologized afterwards saying he knew that wasn't fair of him to ask of his child…those memories haunt me to this day. I never did help him.

Where was my mom? you may be thinking… well, like I said, she was a narcissist and she was busy with boyfriends and taking care of herself.

When my dad was first diagnosed with Alzheimer's I blamed myself for many years. I recall after my dad's diagnosis my mom saying that "he was fine until he had back surgery." I disclosed to my mom then that I used to fake fall asleep in the car so that my dad would carry me. I recall crying and saying that dad's surgery was all my fault. My mom said nothing to me. I was 11 years old. I felt so guilty.

For years I thought that his illness was because of me; I recall one evening when he was carrying me in from the car, he almost dropped me because his back went out. It was shortly after this that he had to have surgery on his back, and then a very short time later he began to slowly lose his brain function. It wasn't until I was in my late teens that I broke down crying to a social worker in dad's hospital, saying that it was "all my fault" that my dad was so ill. I explained about my dad's back surgery, the social worker reassured me that his illness had nothing to do with his back surgery. I recall my mom sitting there expressionless. I would later learn that my dad had a pre-existing back injury from the war.

I learned about my dad's previous back injury from my brother Bob when I was in my 50's. He explained to me how in WW11 my dad, a Sergeant, was blown out of a tank while checking for land mines. His entire platoon was killed, my dad was knocked unconscious and would remain that way for several days. He was flown home and they discovered then that his back was broken. This story was originally told to Bob by our dad.

My childhood was long and when not playing with friends I remember feeling very lonely and isolated. My brothers were all so much older than I was and they weren't around a lot, except Bill, we were seven years apart and we basically grew up together. Bill taught me how to ride my first two-wheeled pedal bike and being a typical older brother, he taught me from the top of a steep hill! I was pedalling along just fine until I realized he had let go and then I lost control and crashed into a tree. We were always playing tricks on one another and getting each other into trouble with our parents, but for the most part we spent a great deal of time together catching salamanders, listening to music, swimming and going for long bike rides. Bill and I have remained close throughout our adulthood and he has always been my protector. When I was about 7 years old, he saved me from nearly drowning, he used to keep the school bullies at bay too.

Nick and I really connected about 25 years ago and we have remained close ever since. We connected after his separation and eventual divorce from his wife. Nick slipped into a deep depression and was suicidal. I spent many weekends with him and counselled him the best I could. I was happy to do this for my brother and I felt needed. He lived in the Vancouver area and I was still living on Vancouver Island. Together we formed a strong bond and while out dancing one night, he met his new partner, a lively and vivacious woman, Laurie. They were co-workers and already knew each other. We all remain close to this day.

At one time, many years ago, Don and I were close both geographically and emotionally. For me, when I see Don now that emotion and those good memories come flooding back. Don, or DJ as he prefers to be called now, is a tender hearted, sensitive and caring man. We don't see much of each other, but without a doubt we love each other dearly. He resides with his wife Mea and as far as I know he is happy and content. We rarely see one another and live hundreds of miles apart.

Because of our age differences we each had different experiences growing up. My brothers talk about times when our mom would be gone for days, leaving them on their own at very young ages. During this timeframe, our mom would be gone with other men. Nick recalls coming home from school one day to find our brother Bill alone and sitting in his high chair. Nick had to stay home and care for him (and Don and Bob) until our mom returned home two or three days later. Their dad would either be gone to work camp or out hunting for meat to feed them. I grew up poor, but my understanding is that their early years were marked as dirt poor and they were all neglected by our mom.

CHAPTER 2

ABUSE AND BROKEN MARRIAGES

The first memory I have of being sexually abused was when I was five years old; I was at my friend *Debbie's house. Her brother *Daryl was 18 and wanted to play hide and seek with us. Only, he changed the rules, him and either Debbie or me would go into the bathroom and count while the remaining girl hid. When it was my turn to "count" with Daryl he forced me to perform fellatio on him. He threatened to beat me if I told. Of course, I told Debbie as soon as I got the chance that day. All I can remember is telling her in whispered secrets and her holding the back door open and telling me to "run home!" I remember running as fast as I could.

When I got home, I told my mom. Indifferently, she replied, "well don't go over there anymore then" I begged my mom to let me go there still, I asked her "what about Debbie?" as even at my young age I knew to fear for her. My mom said not to worry about Debbie and that "whatever you do; do not tell your dad." I didn't tell my dad. I didn't tell anyone again until I was an adult. As a child I would continue to go over to Debbie's house and Darryl was always sent downstairs to work with their parents at their home business. I suspect that Debbie had told her parents.

My mom and I never talked about it again. She would never ask me if I was okay. I never had Debbie to my house as my dad wouldn't allow me to have any friends over, whenever I asked why, he would reply "I don't need to have another damned mouth to feed." I often wonder about Debbie and how her life turned out. I remember how kind her mom was. On cold mornings, she'd warm Debbie's milk for her cereal before putting it in a bowl. She'd stroke her hair and always showed her love to her. At five years old, I remember thinking that I wished I was Debbie.

The second time that I remember being sexually abused was at the age of 8 and it continued until I was 14, only this time when I told my mom she didn't believe me. She said I was making the whole thing up to get attention and that I only thought of it because she had been raped as a child and she thought I wanted to "be like (her)" (sic) By this time my dad had been admitted to hospital as he required around the clock care.

Before he went to the hospital however, I remember hearing my parents arguing, my dad was saying "that's not right for that old man to be spending time with our daughter. Something isn't right here" My mom had replied "she's fine." It's amazing that as ill as my dad was, he still had the sense to know that something was wrong with 76-year-old *Malcolm spending so much time with his young daughter.

I met *Malcolm when I was about 8 years old, he was a family friend and church goer of one of my friend's and classmates, *Donna.

Donna introduced me to *Malcolm at church and then again at his house as he was a fairly close neighbour to her. The sexual exploitation and abuse that I experienced still causes me to have nightmares. To this day, I cannot speak, or write, of the things he did to me without feeling dirty and ashamed.

I can recall vividly the first and the last time that *Malcolm sexually abused me. The first time was on a swing in his back yard. The last time was in his car. I won't go into detail, but I will say that the images in my mind are painful and debilitating.

The sexual abuse I experienced occurred three to four times a week for six years. I would have to go over to his place afterschool. *Malcolm threatened me to go to his place, if I didn't go, he said, he would tell people what I allowed him to do to me. I was just a little girl and I was scared. I blamed myself for the abuse. I thought that I was a bad girl. I never knew that it was Malcolm that was evil. He would drive me home afterwards and he would lie to my parents and tell them that he was teaching me wood work. I recall one Mother's Day he made my mom a beautiful plant stand, he stated to my mom that we had made it together when in reality he had made it himself. In return I had to pay him with sexual favours. He would often kiss me good bye in front of my parents, what they didn't see was that he would stick his tongue in my mouth when he kissed me.

I was still in elementary school, when I became aware that he sexually abused two other girls in my class. He would make them perform sexual acts on one another while he watched. On occasion, I was put in a separate room and he would perform sexual acts on me. I remember crying and feeling so scared. I think one of the girls told her dad about *Malcolm as they hastily moved out of town one week, at least that's what I was told by *Donna.

When I was about 13 years old, I realized that what *Malcolm was doing was wrong. I was still afraid of him. The abuse took on a different nature, instead of him taking me to his garage, he would take me in his car to different remote locations around town, and he would sexually abuse me in his car. He said we had to go for drives because his "...wife was growing jealous of our relationship." (sic) He would always drive me home afterwards and give me a family size Kit Kat bar. Shortly after my 14th Birthday I told *Malcolm that what he was doing was wrong and that I wouldn't come and see him anymore. He became very angry and said that I had to come over or else he would tell my mom that I was a drug addict and that I was trying to blackmail him for money. I told him that she wouldn't believe him. He smiled and said "oh I can make her believe me."

Shortly thereafter, *Malcolm had gotten to my mom and told her that he was "worried" about me being on drugs and that I "may lie" about being sexually abused. My mother believed him. That was the first time I moved out of the house. I went to Prince George, B.C., and lived with my brother Bob, his wife Mona and their three children. My mom cried at the airport when I left, she sobbed "I cannot believe that you'd do this to me" Dejected, I simply walked away.

Like I said, the only reason I believe that the sexual abuse ended when I was 14 was because I had confronted my abuser. I told him what he was doing was wrong. I told him that I was going to tell my mom, he was right when he said that she'd never believe me and that he could convince her otherwise. My mom would continue to converse with the elderly family "friend" while I lived with my brother and his family for about 15 months. I came home then, because my mom said "maybe" I was telling the truth, she couldn't be sure she said.

*Names have been changed

My life in Prince George was good. I went to school, I had chores and I was part of my brother's family. I was treated kindly and with respect and love. I told Mona a little bit about *Malcolm and she said "I believe you Darlene and I love you." Sweeter words had never been spoken to me about the sexual abuse that I had endured.

*Malcolm telephoned my mom shortly after I had moved back home, I was sitting at the kitchen table when I heard my mom say to him "I don't think you should call here anymore now that Darlene's home." She hung up the phone, glared at me and burst into tears saying "you better not be lying" I was devastated.

We would live this way until I was 16 and my mom got a serious boyfriend, he was my boyfriend's dad. I asked my mom if she wanted to live with her boyfriend and she said of course, but that she couldn't because "how would it look" to the community members of our small town, the two of us moving in with our boyfriends?

She had a point, so I offered to move out on my own, she agreed and quickly moved in with her boyfriend. To this day this stuns me, I never thought she'd take me up on my offer. The "deal" was I had to stay in school and I had to support myself. She wouldn't give me a dime. I was in grade 11. I moved in with a friend, she was a couple of years older than me, but I quickly learned that she was overcharging me for the rent. I moved out of this apartment. I broke up with my boyfriend, *Andy, around this time too. *Andy and I had a "normal" teenaged relationship. We were together for a little over a year when we broke up.

I moved in with another girlfriend, we got along well, but then I met a guy. By this time, I had to quit school because I couldn't get enough work after school hours to cover my expenses and go to school. I wasn't allowed to move back home, so in the winter of my grade 11 year I quit school. My mom was furious, my ever-judgemental mom, queried out loud "how will this look?" She still however refused to help me out financially. I cried, she twisted my words and my actions making her the victim and me feeling like a rotten self-centered daughter.

I moved to Edmonton, Alberta with my boyfriend. It was a terrible two-year life lesson for me. He was abusive in every way imaginable; sexually, physically, emotionally and psychologically. I worked and paid our rent, he had a job once shovelling snow, he lasted about 3 days then he quit. The onus was on me to pay our way in life.

I got a job managing a Greek restaurant in Edmonton, Alberta. I was 17 years old. I lied about my age stating that I was 20. I also lied and said I had experience waitressing; I told these lies so that I could get the job. I started working as an assistant manager. My duties included waitressing and managing the staff, eventually I began managing the entire restaurant. I worked hard and with my tips I made enough money to cover our living expenses.

My boyfriend had numerous affairs, when I caught him having one, I left him. I was terrified that he would come after me. He had threatened me in the past; stating that if I ever left him, he would hunt me down and kill me. I left one afternoon pretending to go to work. He didn't know that I had already quit my job. I took a taxi to the airport and waited on standby for a flight that would take me back to B.C. I remember feeling so scared at the airport waiting for what seemed like an eternity, I was able to get a seat on a flight and I made it to Port Alberni. I called him that night and told him that our relationship was over. I felt safe being thousands of miles apart.

Once he realized that I had I left him for good, he came after me and tried to kill me on several occasions; once with a whaling spear (thank God he missed and while he was trying to remove the spear from the wall that it had stuck into, I was able to escape) and many other times thereafter he tried to run me off the road. He went to jail for a year and was ordered out of B.C. for two years following his prison sentence. This punishment was practically unheard of then, it was 1982 and men didn't go to jail for domestic violence, it was after all a "family problem" (sic)

I would have nightmares after we broke up. One of his favourite ways to torment me was when I was in the bath he would come into the bathroom, plug in the radio and hold it over the bath water threatening to drop it in the bath tub, electrocuting me. Other times he would just like to hold my head under water to see how long I could hold my breath. He always laughed at me before, during and after. The sexual abuse was humiliating and he'd dress me up to look like a little girl. I still suffer the trauma of his abuse.

When I returned to B.C., from Alberta at the age of 18 I had nowhere to go, I asked my mom if I could stay with her, she said no, that it still wouldn't look right because she was living with my ex-boyfriend's dad. I pleaded with her saying that my ex wasn't living there, she still said no. I had some savings and rented a basement suite. I applied for Unemployment Insurance (UI) and was turned down because I had quit my job in Alberta to move to B.C., I appealed their decision and explained before a UI appeals board that I had to quit my job in order to leave an abusive relationship. They agreed that I had "just cause" and paid me UI Benefits. I was so relieved. I recall how nervous I was appearing before this panel of two men and one woman. I was all alone. I had to go into detail about the abuse and I also gave them a copy of the police report.

I only received $77.00 a week and it wasn't enough to live on and pay my rent. My mom reluctantly agreed to let me live on her boyfriend's property and she bought a 17-foot travel trailer for me to live in. I lived there for several months. I was allowed to shower in the house and sometimes they'd have me over to the house for dinner and to play Yahtzee or crib. I really liked her boyfriend and we became close friends.

I then met another man, whom I would later marry. We had two beautiful baby girls together. When we first met, we both worked and partied hard. When I got pregnant the partying stopped – for me, but not for him. We lived in poverty.

For about 18 months we lived in a rented trailer in a remote area by the airport in Qualicum Beach, B.C., It wasn't skirted, so when it froze in the winter so did our pipes and we wouldn't have running water. We didn't have cablevision or a phone. It was heated with an oil furnace and we rarely had money for oil. I used to keep the kids in the kitchen and heat the kitchen area by turning on the oven and keeping the oven door open. We had a CB radio for emergencies. The only other person that I knew with a CB radio was my father-in law and he detested me because, he said, I had "trapped" his son into marriage and babies. There were no neighbours, no street lights and no sidewalks, it was a gravel road. I had a cheap umbrella stroller and I can remember walking to the grocery store with my swollen baby belly and my one-year-old down this gravel road for two miles to get diapers and whatever else I could carry. My husband had the car with him in Ucluelet where he worked at a fish plant. He rented a house there with some family and work mates and he lived there while he worked. On his days off, if he had money for gas, he would come home and see me and our eldest daughter. I was pregnant with our second daughter and would give birth to her during this timeframe. I was miserable, lonely and broke. We didn't have garbage pick-up and I used to dump the diapers in the back yard and try and burn them (disposable diapers don't burn). It wasn't long before we had rats in the yard.

I remember my mom came to visit me and my babies, it was a surprise of course because she had no way of contacting me. I burst into tears because, other than my children, I hadn't seen or spoken to anyone in over ten days. I had no food in the house and was almost out of diapers. I begged my mom to take me to her home for a few days. I told her I had no money and no food. She took me home with her and I stayed for five glorious days before she took me and the kids back to our home. My husband came home too and had a paycheque so we had money for food and diapers. One time, my sister-in-law, Marita, came for a visit with my mom. They asked for a cup of tea. I remember that I only had one tea bag left, so I made us each a cup of tea using the one tea bag. They asked for more tea, I burst into tears and said I didn't have any more tea bags and that I had nothing more to offer them. They left shortly afterwards. I was so embarrassed.

It was right around this time that I told my husband that I couldn't live like this anymore. I put our name in for low-cost housing in Port Alberni, I told him that the kids and I were moving there with or without him. He reluctantly agreed to come. If I thought his dad hated me before he really hated me now. He told me I was a terrible person for taking his son out of a "home" and "forcing him" to move into an apartment. He said he'd "never" forgive me and he didn't. He would die almost 35 years later still despising me.

My husband hated our home, whereas I loved it, we had three bedrooms and 1 ½ bathrooms. It was heated, we were warm and comfortable. The housing was big and new. He would spend most of his time out in our shed tying flies for river fishing. We rarely spoke. Months passed, I gave him the choice alcohol or me and the kids. He chose the alcohol, by the time he was ready for change, I was done. It was a tumultuous relationship. He was a messy drunk, he'd pee in the closet or not come home for days. One time when he came home after being gone for a couple of days, I accused him of cheating on me; he punched me so hard in the face that I fell backwards into the closet door, breaking it, and landing on my bottom. I recall another time he came home so inebriated that he threw-up all over himself in our bed. I was done then, but it would take me another six months to end our marriage.

During this six-month time frame, my brother Bill moved in with us. He and my husband worked together for a while. We all got along great and I was sad to see my brother move out and return to Vancouver, B.C.

When our youngest daughter was one years old, our marriage ended. I kept the kids with me and he moved back to his home town of Qualicum Beach, B.C. and the children and I stayed in Port Alberni. He demonstrated an absolute hatred for me and unfortunately took it out on our children, by not seeing them, as he didn't want me to have any free time. To this day he will not speak to me and our children are now in their mid-30's. In short, we were too young to get married and have babies and he liked his alcohol too much. Anyway, it was a very long time ago and after all these years he still despises me. Ironically it should be the other way around I suppose, but it's not.

When my husband moved-out I had no income, when he could, he'd pay me $200.00 a month for child support, but this would seldom happen. I went on welfare and was on it for three or four months. I was so good at balancing a budget that I would have money left over at the end of each month. I hated the stigma of being on welfare and I felt very ashamed when I'd go to the bank and cash my cheque. I felt that the bank tellers looked down upon me and some made negative remarks. I went to the Canada Unemployment Office and they told me that they were just starting a new program and that if I returned to school, I would receive unemployment cheques each month instead of welfare! "Would I be interested" they asked? Would I!

Around this time my mom remarried. She met and married a fantastic man. He was kind, loving and caring. His love was true and he accepted me and my daughters into his heart without question. My mom never had problems meeting men; she was good looking and a master at being the manipulative person she needed to be to get what she wanted and that included men. Men fell head over heels in love with my mom and my new step dad was no exception. They were married for 25 years before he succumbed to congestive heart failure. I loved him dearly and so did my children. He had become my "dad" and filled an empty void for me that my biological father had left behind.

In later years I would discover that my mom never did love him, I found this out after his death when she said to my middle daughter that she only married him for his money. She told this to my daughter while giving her "marital advice." My daughter was devastated, she loved her grandpa and he was her favourite person.

In retrospect this shouldn't really surprise me as when my dad was in the final stages of congestive heart failure his doctor put him in palliative care. My mom and I were told he only had days left to live. In our presence the doctor explained this to my dad. Sadly, he took off his wedding band and handed it to my mom. That's when I knew his life was over as despite how many times my dad had surgery in the past and the many times he was admitted to hospital, he would never ever remove his wedding band, stating to the nurses and doctors that they could "cut it off me when I'm dead, until then this ring doesn't get removed." The significance of him removing his wedding band was not lost on me.

The next day my dad rebounded! He was full of life and when I went to see him, he was sitting on the edge of his bed eating his favourite breakfast, porridge, or "mush" as he called it! My daughters had all come to say goodbye to their favourite person, their grandpa, and one by one they sat alongside him and in private and with the greatest of dignity he talked to each of them about death and dying. My mom on the other hand was furious, she and I met with the doctor and she demanded to know why he was being fed. When he was "supposed to be dying." The doctor, who was quite baffled by my mom's behaviour, stated that my dad had rebounded and he didn't know how long the rebound would last; days, weeks or more and that he "certainly" wasn't going to stop feeding him "madame." My mom angrily said "well I thought he was dying, now I suppose I have to give him his ring back."

My kind hearted step father who loved my mom unconditionally was devastated by my mom's behaviour towards him. She was cold hearted when she offered him his ring back and as I stood there and stared at her in disbelief, he refused the ring and said "you keep it." He barely spoke another word to her thereafter. He died two days later with what I am sure was a broken heart. I stood by his side, holding his hand, and with a tear in his eye I watched him take his last breath. My daughters and I were devastated, whereas my mom barely shed a tear. But I digress..

I decided to return to school. I went back and completed grades 11 and 12 and then I wrote my GED (grade 12 equivalency) test and I passed! I then went to college and got a diploma in business management. All of this was covered by unemployment insurance benefits! They even covered my daycare costs so that I could be in classes.

By then I had met my second husband. If I thought that my previous boyfriend was mean he had nothing on my second husband. We were together for four years. The first year we dated, the second year we lived together and he was my KNIGHT IN SHINING ARMOUR. That was until we got married, he changed on our honeymoon and became a monster. I honestly don't know how I lived through that marriage, but I did for two years. Thankfully we never had any children together.

I don't know how or when his control over me started, but he controlled my every move. He knew how far the grocery store was from our house and he would check the car's odometer when I got home. If I got a good cut of meat, he claimed it was because I was "fucking the butcher." He got home from work every day at 4:40pm and dinner had to be on the table at 4:45 or else. I never had the nerve to disobey and find out what the "or else" meant. I recall making a ham dinner one night, he picked the ham up off the table and threw it in the garbage. He grabbed me by my throat and squeezed and said "I don't eat fucking pig puss!" I never cooked us pork again.

Another time, my mom and my step-dad were due at our house any moment to drop off my daughters, after having spent a weekend together. I don't recall what I had done, but something triggered a rage in him so fierce that he picked me up by my throat and held me against the wall while threatening to throw me out the living room window, landing, he said, on my parent's car. "What would you think about that you dumb bitch?" he yelled. (I could go on and on with daily examples, but I think you get what I mean.)

My mom came to the door, I ran and opened it and I told to her what my husband had done. She looked shocked, but didn't say anything. She came in and I made tea, I whispered to my mom "invite me grocery shopping" she did and her and I were able to get out of the house without incident. I begged my mom to help me, she said she didn't have room for the girls and me nor did she want to get involved. I lit a cigarette and she lectured me on smoking, saying it was a dirty disgusting habit. That lecture went on and on. My mom was good at doling out shame and I was really good at stuffing it inside. I had grown-up shame based and I knew it well. Being a former smoker herself, I would have thought that she would have had a little compassion, but she did not.

I would later get the courage to leave, but it took the kindness of two people that I barely knew, Ken B and the late Nancy M to help me.

Before I moved out, the abuse was horrendous and it was every day. I became so anxious and scared that I catered to his every whim. I wasn't allowed to go anywhere with friends or family. He controlled everything, what I ate and drank and what I wore and who I talked to. He had sexual intercourse with me every night whether I wanted to or not. When I tried to say no, he would reply "I wasn't asking." I would often lay there unresponsive with silent tears rolling down my face, sometimes he would place a magazine over my face and pretend to have sex with the woman on the cover.

He would go out and party nearly every weekend, I would later discover that he had many illicit affairs. From one of his affairs, he contracted crabs. I recall him having intercourse with me one night and rubbing his pubic area into me with such force that it burned. He would later accuse me of giving him crabs (although by some miracle I never got them) and he threatened to throw me out of the house, but because he was a "caring" husband he would "let" me stay. He told me how "lucky" I was, no other man would take that from me. Sadly, I believed him thinking I must have contracted crabs from a toilet seat and gave them to him.

The thought never entered my mind that he was being unfaithful to me.

I only had the courage to leave because my doctor asked me why I stayed with such a monster, I said because I have children to think of. He looked me in the eye and said "…and who's going to raise your children after he kills you? Him?" Shaken to the very core, I left my husband within weeks of that conversation.

I met Ken and Nancy through my little sister Kimmy. Kimmy is a dear friend whom has become my "chosen sister." Nancy was her mom and Ken is her step-father. Kimmy and I have been through so much together and my life would be empty without her in it. I can confide anything to her. We met at a party when she was just 17 and I was 22. Kimmy lived with me and my second husband for a few months. She witnessed his abuse firsthand. She was appalled and would gently tell me that I didn't deserve that kind of treatment. She helped to keep me sane. Kimmy was young and although she witnessed a lot she certainly didn't know about the sexual abuse.

Nancy, Ken and I would later become good lifelong friends as well; celebrating many of life's great adventures!

CHAPTER 3

BACK TO SCHOOL (AGAIN)

So now here I was at the ripe old age of 27, twice divorced, with two little girls to take care of on my own. My mother refused to help me even though she knew most of what I had been through. I had nowhere to go, and then a loving angel of a woman, Nancy, and saint of a man, Ken, took me and my two children into their home where we would live off and on for about six months; I tried going back to my marriage, but it didn't work, he continued to cheat and be abusive. We tried marriage counselling, but the counsellor told me that he couldn't help us because my husband was not being honest. I asked him what I should do. With a deep sigh he replied, "I've never said this to a client before but if you were my daughter, I would pack you and the children into my truck and drive you as far away from this man as possible. I'm afraid that if you stay with him, he will kill you." His words impacted me greatly and that's when I left my husband for good.

This brave and kind couple took us in, they didn't even know us, like I said I was friends with their daughter Kimmy. Ken and Nancy would not accept any money from me for room and board. I only had to chip in a very small amount for groceries.

I was able to get two high paying part time jobs. I worked hard and eventually I got us our own basement suite to rent and about a year later I decided to go back to school! I took out a student loan, upgraded my English studies and began a long, tedious and sometimes frightening four-year university bachelor's degree in the social work program at the University of Victoria. It would take me six years to complete the four-year program.

While working at one of my jobs, in the food services section of our community hospital, I walked into a hospital room to deliver a food tray to a patient. I stopped dead in my tracks. The patient was *Malcolm. He laid there and didn't show any sign that he recognized me. He sat up and said "hello dear" and without a word from me, I placed his food tray on his table. On the chair beside his bed was a pillow. I don't know how long I stood there staring at that pillow, it may have been minutes or perhaps only seconds. All I recall now is thinking I could put that pillow over his face and smother him. I quickly left his room without saying a word in response to his greetings. That experience terrified me. How could I even pause and think about doing something like that? All the years of abuse came flooding back and I quickly stuffed it down.

So now here I am back in school doing university level transfer credit courses at our local community college! (I would do this for two years before officially transferring my studies to the University of Victoria's distance program.)

My girls and I had a good life, we were poor, but I made sure that they never wanted for anything. We played games to help them with their school work, we got two cats and life was carefree. We did our homework together and had quiet time doing this from 6:00-7:00 every night. I had to let one of my jobs go, it was shift work and I couldn't do the night shifts with the kids. For most of their lives, their father was an absentee dad, they didn't need an absentee mom too. As luck would have it, the house we were living in sold and we had to move. Fortunately, I found another basement suite that I could afford and we moved to our new home.

Like our previous suite this one also had two bedrooms. Again, the girls each got a bedroom and I slept on the couch that made out to a hide-a-bed. I desperately wanted my daughters to have as "normal" a life as possible. I left my second job and took out another student loan so that I could study full time. We would live this way for two years. I dated a fellow casually. Then I met my future soul mate, Rob, my forever love.

CHAPTER 4

SOUL MATES

Rob and I were acquaintances through a mutual friend. We fast became friends before we became lovers. He was kind and generous to me and most importantly to my daughters. We dated for a little over a year and then we moved in together in a house that Rob purchased. Initially, and for me, moving in together was for a huge financial relief and for protection. Rob took care of the home-owner expenses and we split the costs associated with groceries and the utilities. For the first time in my life, I wasn't poor! I say I moved in for protection because it was at that time that I fell victim to a stalker.

I was working at a deli in a grocery store in our community. It was normal of course to have regular customers. This one male customer in particular turned out to be anything but normal. He was an older gentleman, about 20 years my senior, and I can recall he usually came in about five minutes before our store closed on Friday evenings. One Friday evening I said to him "oh here's my last-minute customer, now I know it's almost time to close" we both laughed and apparently that's all it took. He would later be diagnosed as having *erotomania* (a delusion that another person is in love with them). As I understood it, erotomania is a common diagnosis of stalkers whom normally are afflicted with this mental disorder when stalking celebrities. I am NOT for one second inferring that I was a celebrity I am simply stating that this type of occurrence is rare for that of a regular person in a regular situation. That is, celebrities are popular and are stars in movies etc., they have a large social audience, so that if someone (a stalker) in the population happens by chance to see the celebrity (and is predisposed to) then erotomania may occur. This certainly couldn't happen in a small town in Port Alberni to a lowly deli clerk?! But it did. The more I tried to avoid him the more aggressive his behaviour became. It got to the point where he had planned our wedding and had given invitations to his co-workers. I had had a peace bond placed on him and he apparently posted the peace bond on top of our wedding invitation on a cork board at his work with the caption "women!" and advising that our wedding was postponed.

Needless to say, the police and the courts were involved. For our safety, we moved in with Rob at that time. At one point, the stalker mailed a movie script to the University of Victoria's (UVIC) media department inquiring if they wanted the rights to "our movie" referencing that it could be a sequel to the Hollywood movie "Fatal Attraction" UVIC was so alarmed that they contacted the Port Alberni police (Royal Canadian Mounted Police; or RCMP) and reported the incident.

Myself, I was terrified. I contacted my children's school and ensured that no one was to pick them up from school except me. Rob's brother, Richard, who lived in the Vancouver area contacted a psychologist at the University there (UBC) he did this on my behalf and to see how he could better help me. I met with the psychologist, as Richard had pre-arranged, and he gave me advice on stalkers; as this was a field that he specialized in. He counselled me to not have any contact with the offender, stating that no matter what I did or what I said the offender would misconstrue it to his advantage.

This was a very scary time in my life. I didn't know to what lengths he would go to "to have" me. Would he abduct me? Lock me up somewhere? Would he abduct my children? He was so delusional that he would tell his work mates stories about "our" weekends together. His stories would always include images of my daughters. He would write me letters, that were anywhere from 25-30 pages long, professing his love for me. A few years later, the offender would succumb to cancer.

Rob, the children and I got along well. Rob has an amazing family. They are close and enjoy spending a lot of time together. Each of them welcomed the girls and me into their family with open arms. For Rob, this was "normal" for me this was extremely foreign. His parents had been school aged friends and partners, they married in their twenties and stayed married. They had four children together. There was no cheating or abuse; physical, emotional, sexual or psychological. For each of them this was a normal life, for me this was unheard of. They had family vacations, they had dinners together, they all gathered together over the holidays and they all got along. Sure, there would be little arguments here and there, but that was it. I felt like I didn't belong, not by them, but by me.

They sincerely wanted to know about my past life. Well, let's see, how's this for a sell; I am 27 years old, a single mother of two, twice divorced and a high school drop-out...and yet they all still welcomed and accepted me into their lives. Rob's parents were retired school teachers, they had worked their whole lives at one profession! They had life long friends. Rob had a grandma. Nobody had any "issues" and yet they accepted me. To this day,

I am still dumbfounded by that. I had never before <u>not</u> been pre-judged, it was surreal. I was, and am still, in awe of this family.

Rob and I fell in love. I had long since left my job at the deli. We decided to have a baby together and I had my tubal ligation reversed. We tried for three years to have a baby, the first pregnancy was ectopic and the second was a miscarriage.

The ectopic pregnancy nearly cost me my life. Thankfully I had a skilled, caring and compassionate gynaecologist who was able to repair and rebuild my damaged tube so that I would eventually be able to carry a baby to term. Having an ectopic pregnancy and then a miscarriage a year later was so very upsetting for Rob and I. Together we mourned the loss of our unborn babies.

I was still going to school and because I wanted to give something back to my community, I was volunteering at the local police station as a victim services worker. Through a practicum via the University of Victoria, I was hired at the Crown Counsel Office as a victim services caseworker, working with victims and witnesses of serious crime. It was at this time that an 11- year-old girl in our community would fall victim to a brutal rape and murder. I worked with that family for about four years; establishing a professional relationship; first through the police investigation as a volunteer worker then through the court system as the crown's caseworker (after an in-depth police investigation, the offender was identified via DNA and later convicted of murder).

Our small community of Port Alberni all grieved the loss of this little girl. She was taken so tragically and grievously and the shock and pain was felt by everyone that knew her. For me, working with the little girl's parents, her sister, the grandparents, aunts, uncles and many close friends of the family while liaising with the police, crown and media was challenging to say the least. I would work long days and into the evenings spending my time helping the family cope and help them process through the steps of the legal system. I attended her funeral with the parents and other immediate family. She was a well-known little girl who spent a lot of her time at the ball field and playing hockey. This experience helped me to grow as a professional. As a mother of an 11-year-old girl myself, I was impacted greatly. I suffered many sleepless nights and had nightmares. I had to console my own daughters while at the same time balance my time with the victim's family, my schooling and my work.

It was during this timeframe that I became pregnant and would give birth to a beautiful baby girl. This would be Rob's first biological child and my third. My older girls already had accepted Rob as their step-father and referred to him as dad. My older girls were 12 and 13, by the time their baby sister was born.

Not long after our daughter was born, Rob and I had relationship problems. He had started his own Heavy Duty Mobile Mechanic company and worked in camp for two weeks at a time and then would come home for a week, absolutely exhausted. I had helped him start his company. I spent over 30 hours writing his business plan. Together we presented his business plan to the unemployment investors board where his plan and funding for same was approved.

I was still in school, finishing the last leg of my bachelor's degree, I had a toddler, two teenaged daughters, I did Rob's books and I worked part time at the Crown Counsel Office. I was also exhausted. I remember explaining this to Rob, his response was "quit your job then." My response was to distance myself from him and his family. My "job" as stressful as it was, was my only adult time reprieve. I took up golfing and spent a lot of time with my girlfriends. Rob and I became further distant. I was heart-broken at his response. I was also angry. For me this was the beginning of the end of our relationship.

As fate would have it, my job at the Crown Office ended shortly after I completed my Bachelor's Degree. (But I did it! I held a B.S.W., from the University of Victoria.) The provincial government decided that this program (Crown Victim services) was no longer required and I was designated as "redundant." As you can imagine, for someone with trauma issues being declared redundant was heart wrenching and something I took very personally. I fell into a deep depression. Our youngest daughter was just over 2 years old, putting our oldest girls at 14 and 15 years old.

With my degree, I was able to apply for and eventually became a probation officer with community corrections.

In the meantime, Rob and I went to see a couple's counsellor. Together and through lots of hard work, we were able to work out our differences and we fell in love again. The kind of head over heels, warm and fuzzy, safe and secure kind of love. Most importantly we discovered we were soul mates in the truest sense of the word. Our love continues to grow and blossom. We married in 2004 after having been together for 13 years. Our wedding reception was fun, we had all our friends and family and it was a party to remember!

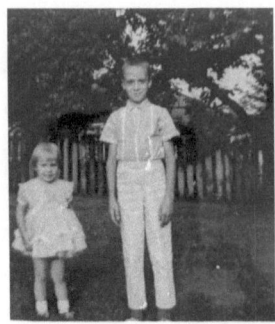 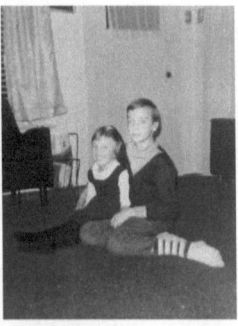 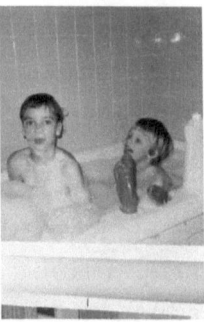

These are photos taken of Darlene and Bill. Ages unknown.

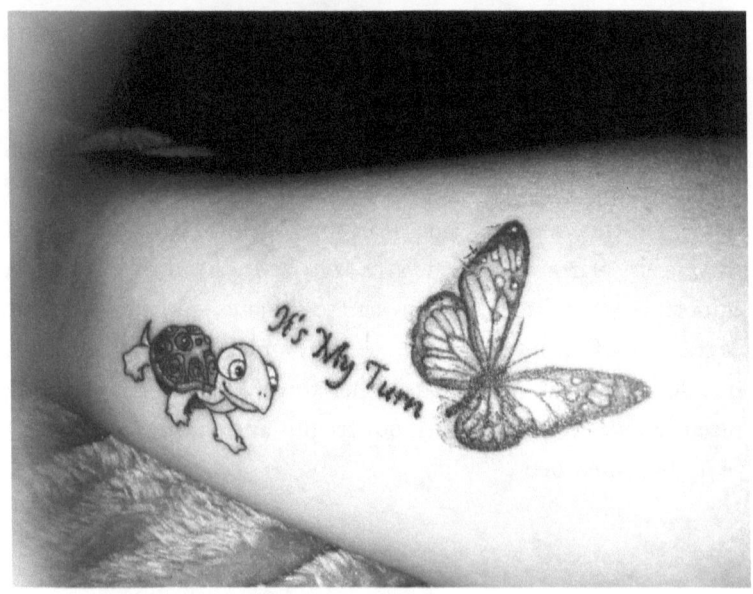

This photo is of Darlene's tattoo. The turtle signifies a slow and steady pace, the butterfly new life and "It's My Turn" to take care of me. This tattoo was created and inked by Darlene's nephew.

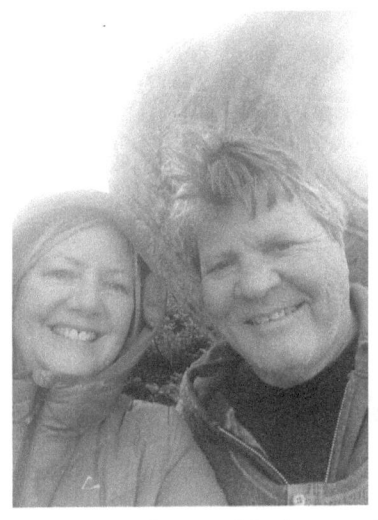 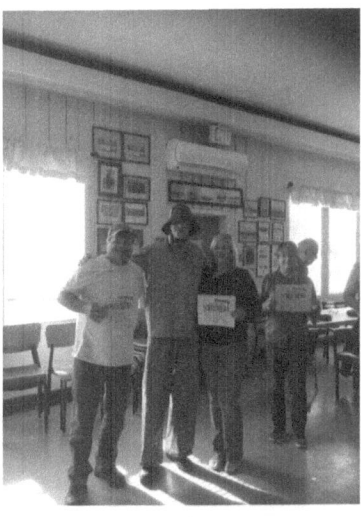

Darlene and Rob motorhome journey 2019/2020
This photo was taken in New Foundland where Darlene and Rob were "screeched in" to become honary "Newfies"

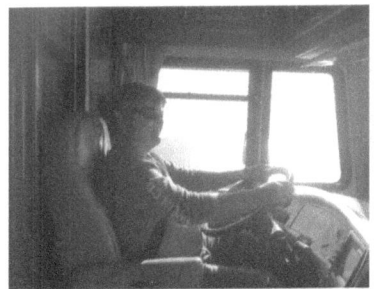 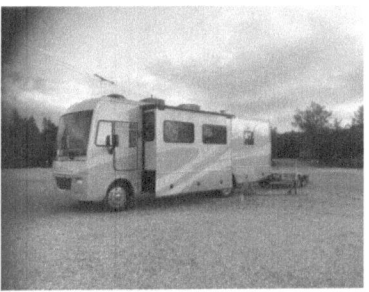

Rob driving the motorhome across Canada in 2019
Our motorhome for our seven-month journey

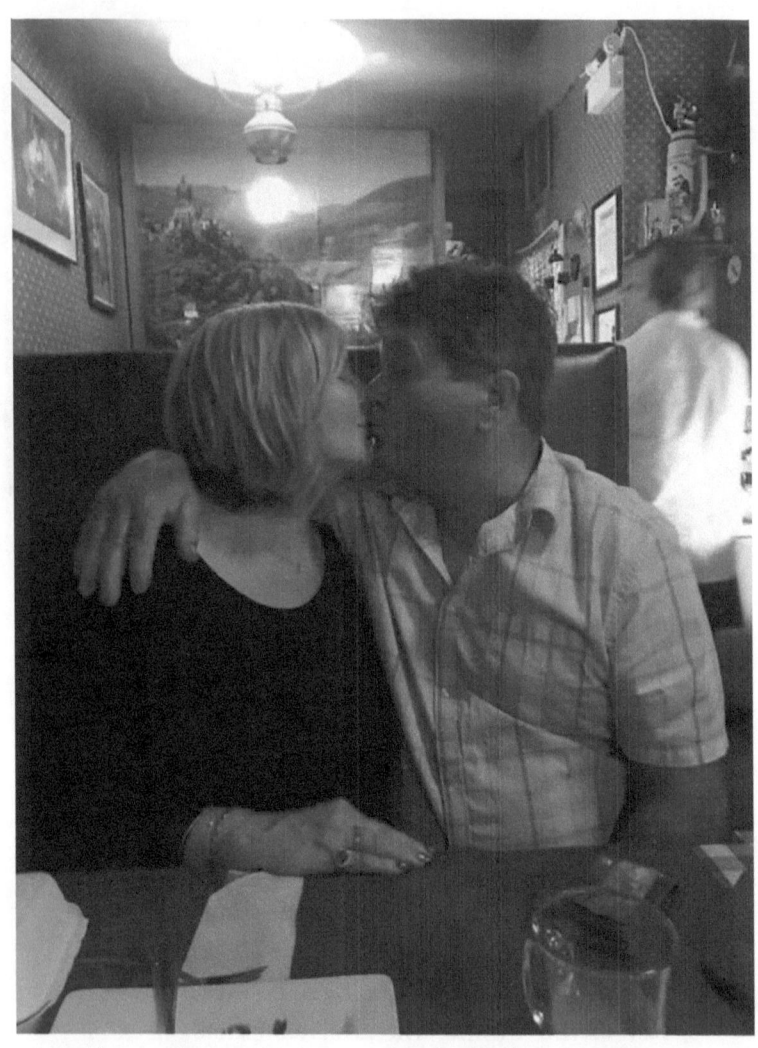

Photo taken at Darlene and Rob's favourite restaurant
Sharing a kiss in Port Alberni.

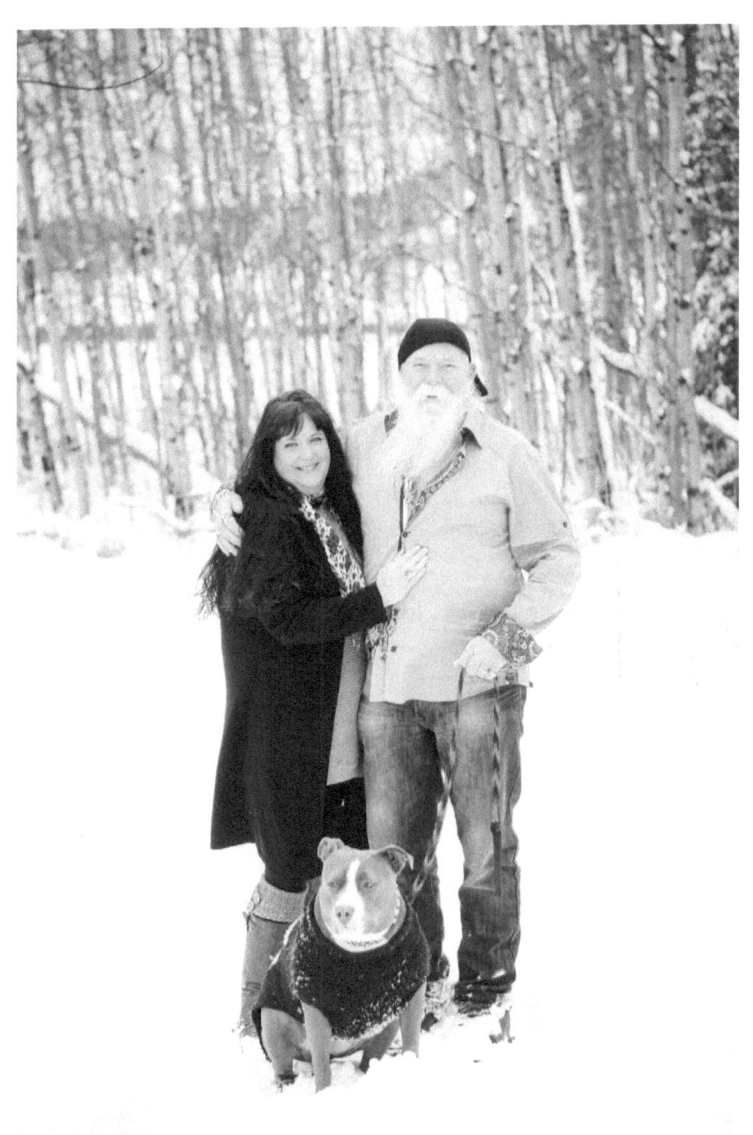

Darlene's brother Don, his wife Mea and their dog

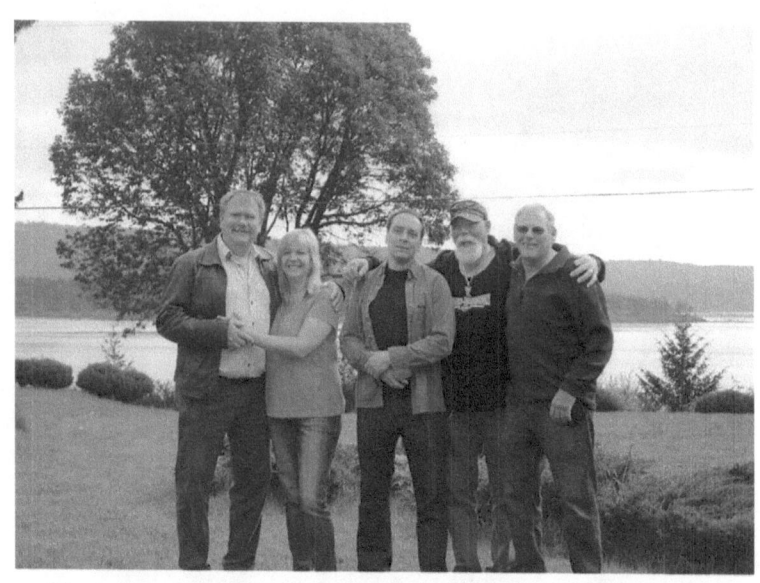

This photo was taken at the last sibling get together in 2014
Left to right; Bob, Darlene, Bill, Don and Nick

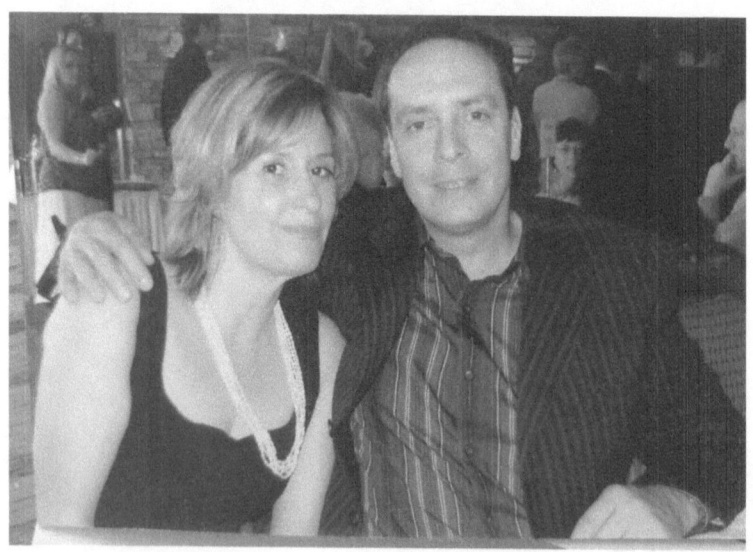

Darlene's brother Bill & his late wife, Lorna

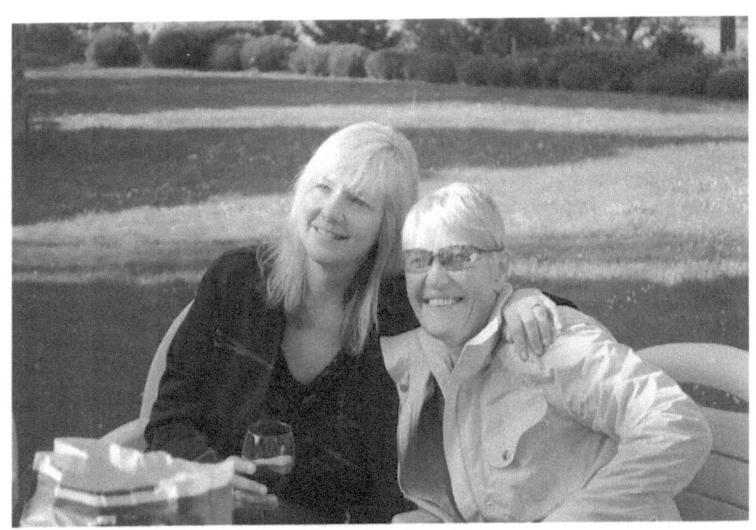

Darlene and sister-in-law Mona (2014)

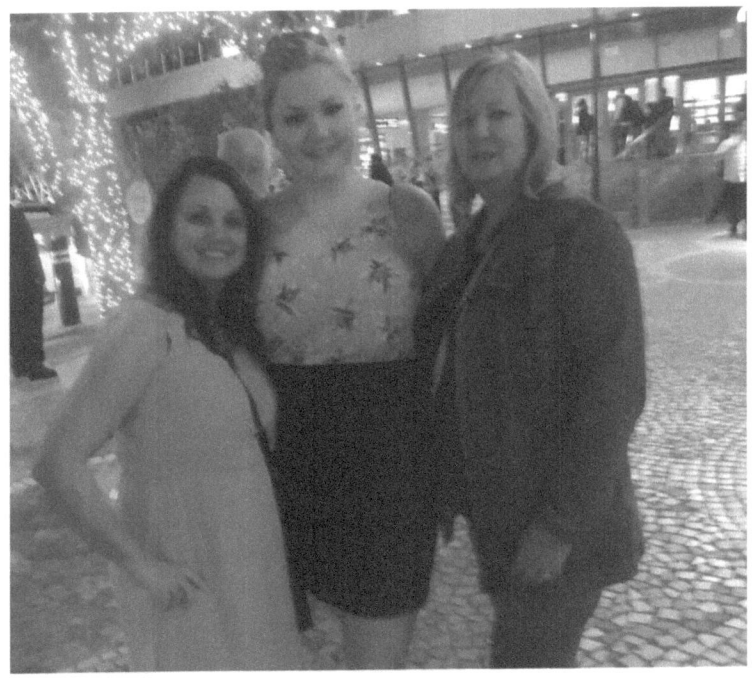

left to right; Kimmy, Elisabeth & Darlene in Vegas

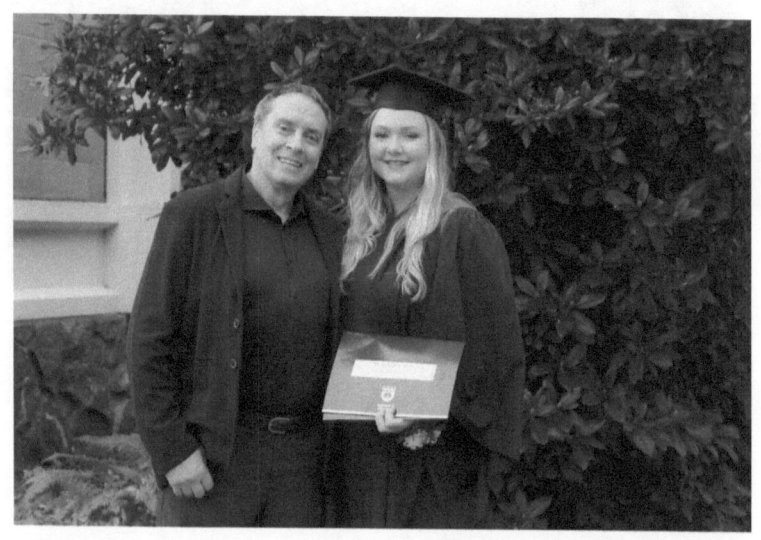

Bill & Elisabeth, photo taken at Elisabeth's grad from UVIC

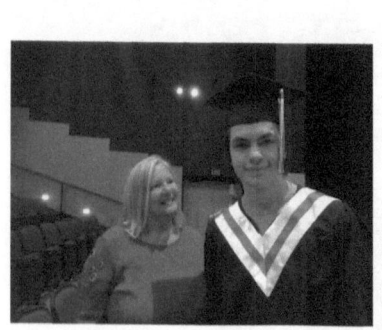 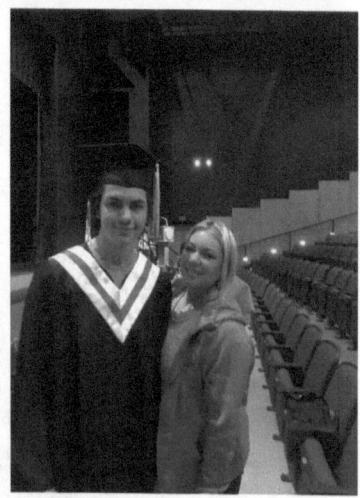

This photo was taken @ Jordan's
grade 12 grad with Nana (Darlene)
Jordan and Darlene's eldest daughter Christine

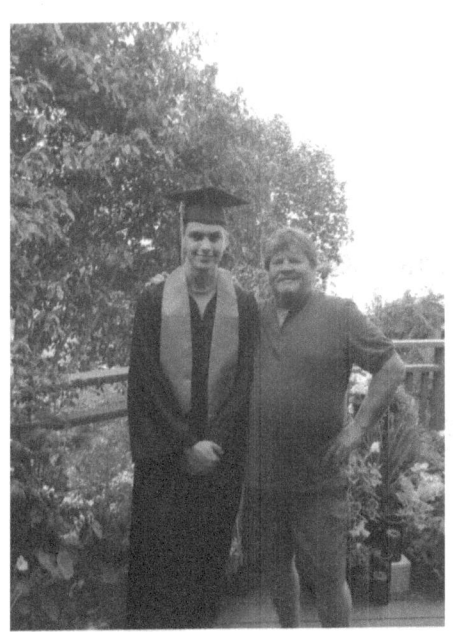

Jordan and his papa (Rob).

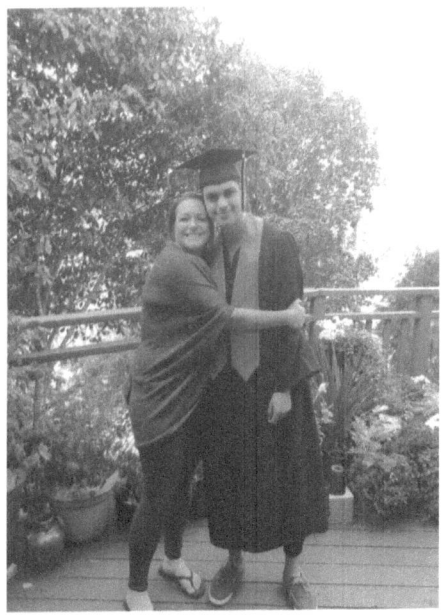

Jordan and Darlene's middle daughter Lisa.

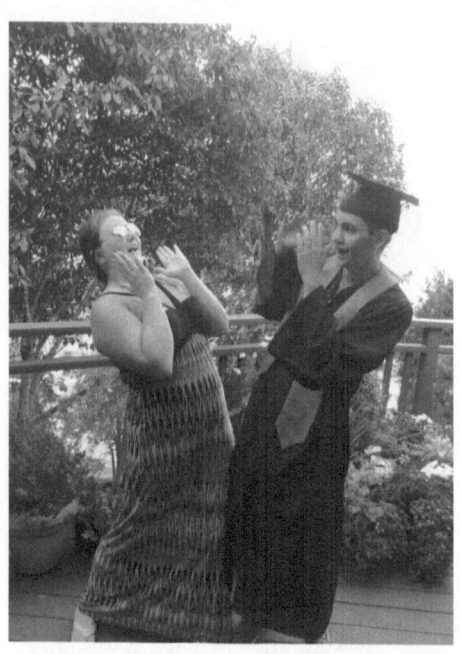

Jordan and Darlene's youngest daughter Elisabeth

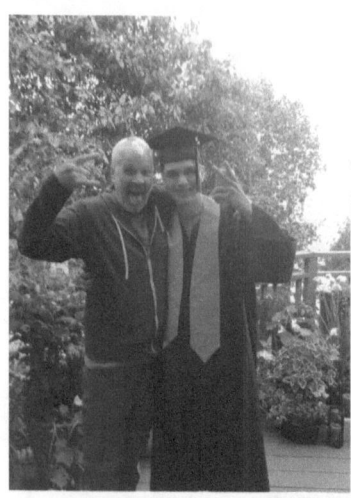

Jordan and his great uncle Richard (Rob's brother)

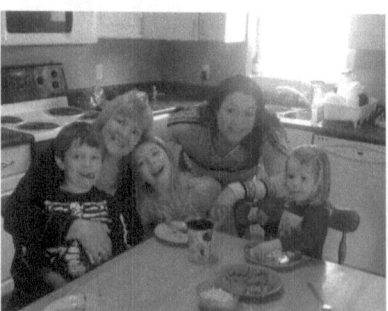

Darlene's grandchildren, left-to right; Owen, (Darlene), Makayla, (Lisa) and Molly

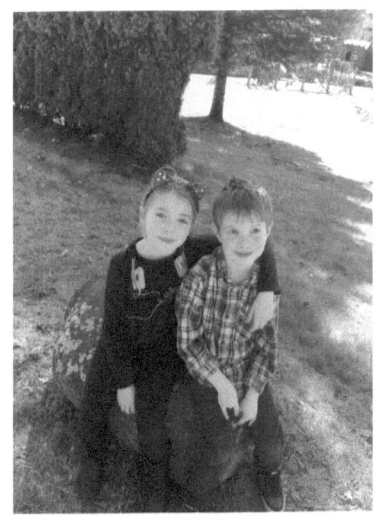 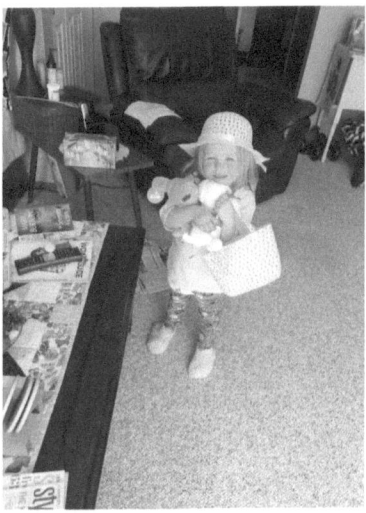

Left to right, Makayla and Owen
Molly

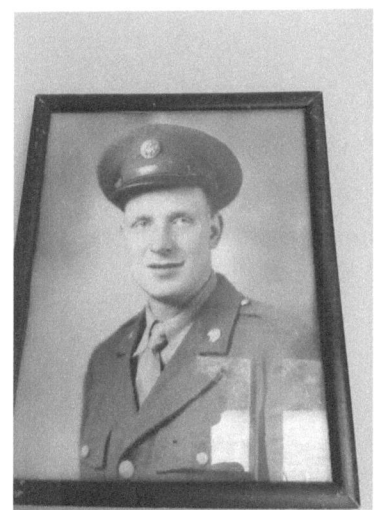 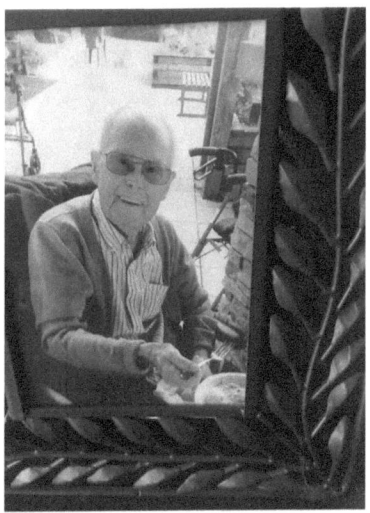

This photo was taken in WW11, (left) Darlene's dad as a soldier
Darlene's step father Bob Wilson

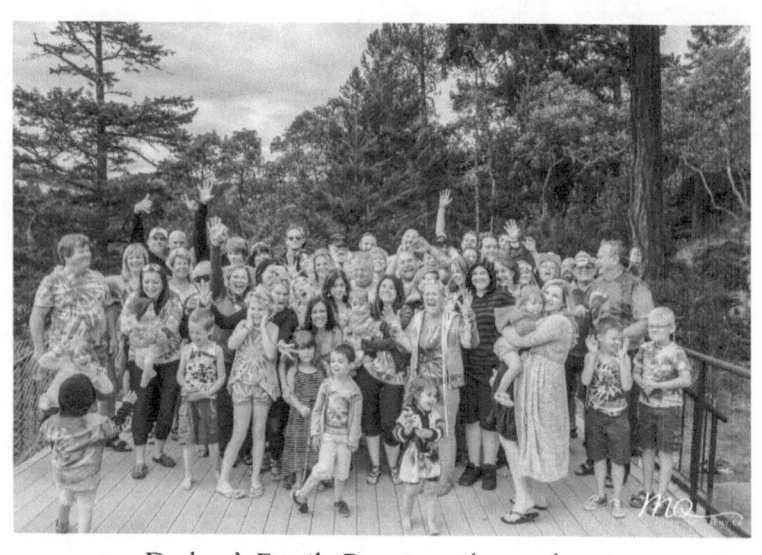

Darlene's Family Reunion, photo taken @
Bob and Mona's in Sooke, BC

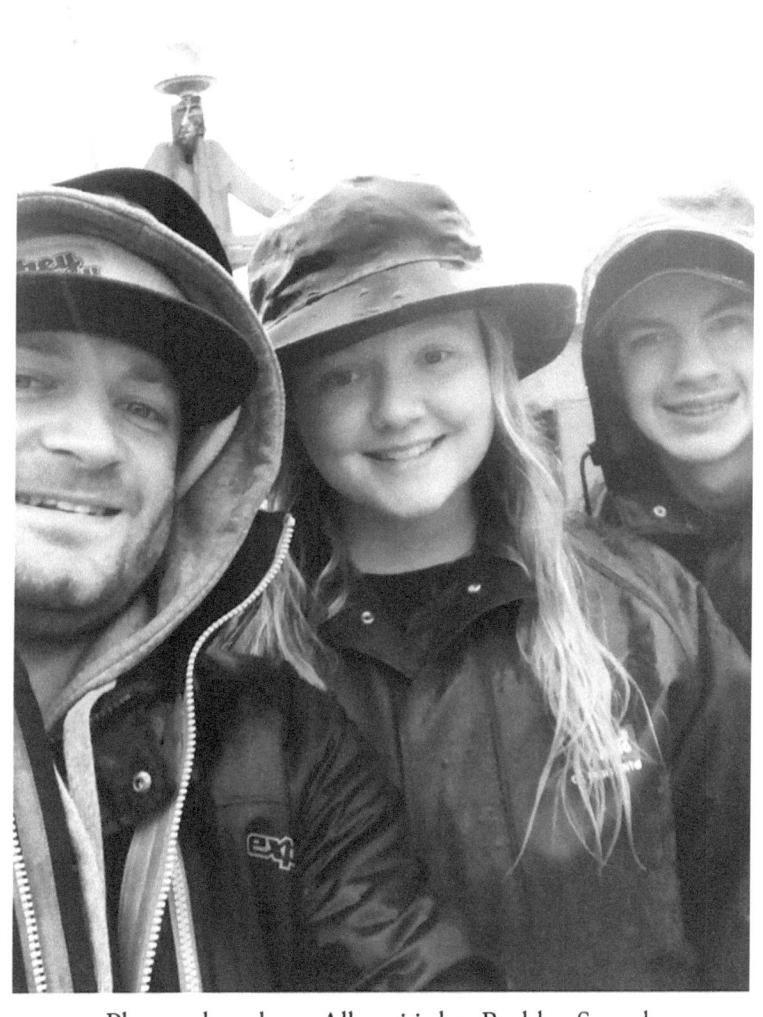

Photo taken down Alberni inlet, Barklay Sound.
Phil, Elisabeth and Jordan on our boat

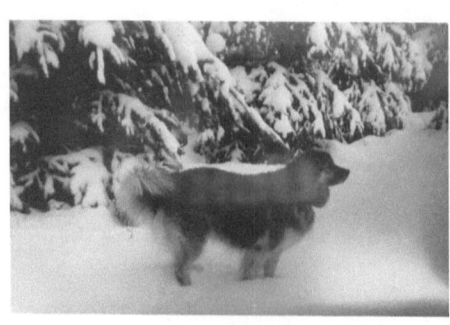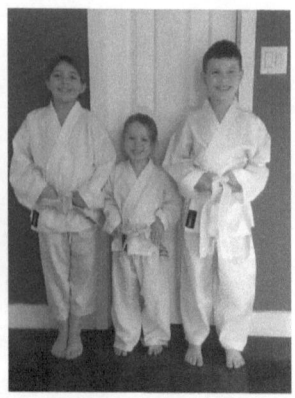

Our dog Mia, one of the last photos we have of her. Makayla, Molly and Owen, ready for jui jit so

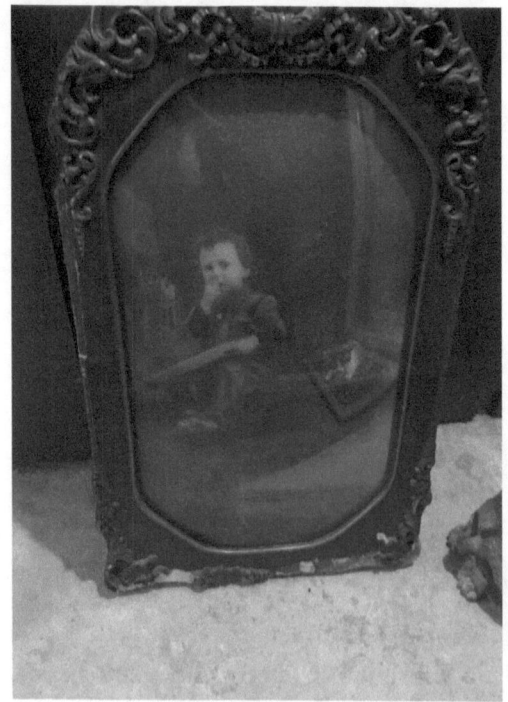

This photo was taken of Darlene's mom as a little girl. Age unknown. Shortly after the photo was taken, she said that she beat the kitten to death with the board she was holding.

CHAPTER 5

RAISING TEENAGE DAUGHTERS

Now, this is where I need to pause and back up in time a little. My eldest daughter was born in 1984. In 1997 and right around her 13th Birthday she changed. A lot. My amazingly perfect and sweet little girl discovered drugs, sex and skipping school. For the very first time as a parent, I was at a complete loss as what to do to help my daughter. I went to counselling. I read her diary. I sought out self-help books. I sought out family and friends; no one and nothing could help me help her. I took her to a pediatrician, he prescribed anti-depressants. I took her to a community-based drug and alcohol counselling centre and counselling at her high school. Nothing seemed to help. I was at my wits end. Rob tried everything too. He tried talking with her. We tried tough love. We tried kindness and soul searching. The more we did, the more she rebelled. She went to the Ministry for Children and asked them to place her in foster care or put her on welfare so she could live on her own. Fortunately, we met with a compassionate social worker that agreed that our daughter should be home with us, just because she didn't want to follow reasonable and realistic house rules, did not garner her the right or the privilege to move out of the family home. Her behaviour affected the whole family. Her then 13-year-old sister, also went into counselling to try and process what her sister was doing to our family. Essentially our eldest daughter's antics was destroying our family dynamic.

Eventually, and at the age of 16, she met a young man and she got pregnant. This young man was horribly abusive to her in every way imaginable. Yet, she stayed with him for a few years thinking and praying that if she "loved him enough" he would change. I honestly don't know how she lived through that relationship, but she did, she even stayed in school and graduated her grade 12 year.

We would see her battered and bruised body and we would go crazy inside. I confronted him more times than not, I was so angry I could have killed him. I have never been filled with such a deep-seated hatred, but to see your child as a victim of domestic violence is absolutely gut-wrenching. She barely escaped with her life. He would eventually go to jail and he was prohibited from entering onto Vancouver Island for two years following his jail sentence. There is a restraining order in place preventing him from contact for 99 years.

My daughter did however bless us with a beautiful grandson. For that we remain eternally grateful. I wish I could say that our daughter's life got better or easier for her, but it did not. She would continue to experience domestic violence well into her mid 30's. We believe her to be in a non-abusive relationship now. We pray. Our relationship is distant, but we love each other a lot. Just before publishing this memoir, we learned that our daughter was indeed in another physically and emotionally abusive relationship. She has left him and charges for assault are against him. I am left heart broken and angry.

Our middle daughter was easy to raise; she caused us no problems, did well at school, did her chores, loved her baby sister and enjoyed family time; cooking, boating, fishing and down at our float cabin in the Barkley Sound. She was funny and talented. She loved to create and was artistic and quirky. She was the peace keeper. In hindsight I should have done more for her. I should have explained that she didn't need to be a perfectionist. She was close with Rob too and they did a lot of fishing together and with friends. I should have spent more time with her and less with her oldest sister. Motherhood is so much simpler in hindsight. They say the child you worry about the least is the one you should worry about the most. It's true. I believe that she could have benefited from a more "hands on" mom. Despite all this or maybe because of this, she grew into a well-respected young lady in our community. She married at 25 and has three of the most amazingly wonderful children. They melt our hearts and every heart that knows them. Unfortunately, our daughter's marriage would end in divorce ten years later. However, her and her ex-husband co-parent together, have a heartwarming friendship and always, always put their children's needs first. We couldn't be prouder.

Our youngest daughter is also a blessing and was easy to raise. She is now in her early twenties, lives with her boyfriend on the lower mainland, works at a forensic psychiatric clinic and is in the process of obtaining her Master's degree in Counselling Psychology. She has a ragdoll cat that she adores and is completely committed to. She has devoted parents, has lived a life of privilege and has never wanted for anything. She was also impacted by her eldest sister's behaviour and they continue to have a strained relationship. This is very sad and disheartening for our family.

As a mother I love all my children equally and to see my eldest child left out of both of her sister's lives is indeed heartbreaking. Change needs to happen with them, but it is not something I can fix. This is something that I have learned only recently. I have an obsessive-compulsive personality and to step back and do nothing is ever so challenging for me. My husband is more accepting of this than I am. Thank God. One thing that has helped me is the *serenity prayer*, that reads, in part:

> **God grant me the serenity to accept the things**
> **I cannot change,**
> **the courage to change the things I can and the**
> **Wisdom to know the difference.**

CHAPTER 6

MY MENTAL HEALTH

I worked as a probation officer from 2002 to 2016. I underwent a lot of training so that I would eventually work with high risk, domestic violent and sexual offenders. I believed that in working with offenders that I would be helping victims of crime. I believed that in addressing the criminal offender's risks, that together we could reduce the risk of recidivism and thus help societies victims.

My work was stressful. I took on a lot, I volunteered in a research project for strategic interventions addressing criminal offender's thoughts, behaviours and attitudes. I believed that I was good at my job. I was passionate and, like all good obsessive-compulsive people, I was entrenched in my work. I worked in isolated communities on the west coast of Vancouver Island including several Indigenous communities.

I believed that I was helping and working with offenders to change their attitudes and thus their behaviours. I worked, alongside my colleagues, and played the role of their coach. I worked with upper management, as well as, the Federal Corrections Department whom was responsible for and the creators of this research initiative, all the while I was carrying a heavy caseload of medium and high-risk offenders. Then I volunteered to receive training to address the criminal thinking of female offenders. Part of my training would involve running a program for this offender type and offering them tools and other life skills.

In short, I burned out. I suffered migraines, developed PTSD like symptoms, fibromyalgia, major depressive disorder and suffered from high anxiety. As a result, I was placed on long term disability where I remain at today. I am on high doses of medication, see a therapist, and I see a psychiatrist who manages my meds and my behaviours. I also see my family doctor regularly and his help and support have been instrumental in my path to recovery. My husband has remained at my side and he has been supportive and kind. He has been my rock.

For me, having to take some time off of work was a very humbling experience. At first, I just thought that I needed a week or two to regain my momentum. I didn't realize just how unwell I was. I certainly didn't think I needed a therapist or a psychiatrist, but I did and I still do. So far in my therapy, I have only touched upon some of my history and some of my work place trauma.

A few months before I left work, I found that I could get teary and cry easily, whereas, before I would not have shown any vulnerability. In fact, the more "twisted" some of my case files were the more I would joke around with my colleagues. I had some files that were so severe that I would not share the details with my colleagues because I was trying to protect them from my nightmares. In short, I didn't want them to also be traumatized. I didn't think that I needed to seek counselling or therapy because I was proud, I was a professional and I could handle anything, or so I thought. I was so wrong, in actuality, it made me mentally unwell. I was deeply impacted and affected. I urge anyone in a helping role or an enforcement position to seek out help, don't let pride get in your way. It is not a weakness to seek help. In hindsight

I believe it to be a strength to reach out to others. I have tried to instill this in my daughters, particularly with my youngest child as she pursues and works in a therapeutic role with others impacted by crime; both offenders and victims alike.

I am now on permanent long-term disability and continue to struggle with PTSD, Migraines, Fibromyalgia, Major Depressive Disorder and Anxiety. I am on a long list of medications to help me cope with these disorders and the trauma associated with it, the medication along with therapy is helping, but I know I have a long road ahead, but most importantly I now know that I am not alone in my recovery.

My mom, now 92 years old, is in a long-term care facility. She continues to manipulate and mess with my head. I cannot stop seeing her however because despite it all, she is my mother and I believe that I should continue to care for her even though she has never cared for me. I am not being a martyr; I do love her and I will miss her when she dies. I will not miss her meanness however. I saw a therapist who believed that I would not begin to heal unless and until I stopped seeing my mom. He was baffled as to why I continued to visit her, and he only knows a small portion of her narcissism. In my opinion, I think that if I did not visit with her, I would be consumed by guilt and that would neither benefit nor help me to heal. I am doing my best to keep our visits short and talk about mundane things. Mostly we talk about her health. She is immobile, incontinent and legally blind. She is moved on a sling from bed to toilet to motorized wheelchair. She is post stroke, has congestive heart failure and is riddled with osteoarthritis and osteoporosis, cognitively she is totally "with it" and I believe that's punishment enough.

Two of my four brothers have nothing to do with our mom. They have zero contact. Part of me wishes that they would connect with her so that Bill and I didn't have to carry all of the responsibility. However, there is another part of me that is envious of them. Sometimes I wish that I could close the door on having contact with my mom, but I simply cannot. Bill and I have grappled with this decision. Neither of us understand why we continue to have contact with our mom, but we do. Our eldest brother Nick calls her weekly and visits her once or twice a year, but he lives off of Vancouver Island and has the rationale and "excuse" (?) not to visit with our mom so often, mostly because of distance, but also because he is in poor physical health himself.

Very recently, my brother Bill decided to stop having contact with our mom. It was not a decision that he made easily. He phoned our mom and told her some of the reasons why he is not wanting contact with her. I respect and admire his decision.

To better understand my mom's meanness, and prior to her living in a long-term care home, one time my mom was in the hospital after suffering a fall. I had been visiting her daily for weeks, making the hour-long drive from Port Alberni to Nanaimo to ensure she was being taken care of and that she was ok. On one such occasion I explained that I wasn't going to stay long (normally I spent a couple of hours with her) stating that I was tired and wanting to go home. My mom was mad. I knew that look, I remembered it from my childhood. Her eyes would actually change colour from brown to black. Deep down I knew she was going to say something mean, but I never imagined she would be so cruel. I was filled with dread and apprehension. She looked me in the eye and carefully and slowly pronouncing each word said: "oh, I never introduced you to my new roommate, his name is <u>Malcolm,</u> you know that name don't you Darlene? <u>Malcolm?</u>" and then she smiled her mean smile.

(*Malcolm was the name of my sexual abuser from when I was 8 to 14 years old).

I was speechless. Under shaky legs I left her and went to the parking lot, and after finding my car, I climbed inside and burst into tears. I sobbed all the way home. I was 50 years old and cried like a baby. I was devastated. How could my own mother hurt me in this fashion? It was unfathomable.

Shortly thereafter, I began experiencing night terrors. In the first instance I awoke and saw a six- foot-tall cricket standing at the end of our bed. The cricket had its arms folded, glasses on the end of its nose and was staring down at me in judgement. I asked out loud "what do you want?" it never replied it just stared at me. In other instances, I would wake up in the night and see giant spiders falling from the ceiling onto our bed. I also saw large poisonous snakes floating in the air around me. I knew they weren't real, but I was scared. I would swat at them and try and make them go away. My husband would wake up and hear me talking to these imaginative creatures.

My doctor referred me to a psychiatrist. He, in turn, adjusted my meds and referred me to a therapist. The experience was terrifying.

Interestingly I would later pay a visit to my mom, as I was talking to her, I looked up and saw her sitting staring at me, arms folded, glasses on the end of her nose judging me. I thought to myself, "oh my God, you're the Cricket.."

This was monumental to me. I finally, after all these years, understood that my mom <u>always</u> cast judgement upon me and it was never ever positive, she would always find something to say to me that was spiteful and hurtful.

Much later, my mental health would also take on another entity – a gambling problem.

I started on-line gambling in April of 2020. My husband and I had just returned home from a seven-month journey in our motorhome. We had travelled across Canada and the U.S.A. It was a trip of a lifetime and my husband and I became even closer.

Our vacation was in our newly purchased motorhome that we had bought second hand from a neighbour. This trip was something that we had dreamed of since early in our relationship. It was a wonderful experience and like I said it brought us even closer together. As fate would have it, the timing of our trip could not have been better.

We came home a week early because of the global pandemic; COVID-19. I was bored, I was home alone a lot, I was lonely, I had always been lucky in Casinos…I have a whole host of reasons why I began online gambling, but I have zero reason as to why it took hold of me, but it sure did. I started off slowly and carefully, but by the last two months I was gambling a lot of money. I lost a lot. I kept chasing those losses and sometimes I'd win, but it was never ever a big enough win, I wanted more and more and more. I was chasing the losses, determined to "win big" and pay off my debt and have enough to buy my husband a new truck and me a new car.

When I realized I was chasing the losses it was then that I stopped gambling. I realized I had a problem. I took an online risk assessment, 1-5 means "maybe" you have a problem or are at least on the verge, the highest score you can get is a 27, I scored 16. The result? I was a "pathological" or "compulsive" gambler. WOW. How in the hell did that happen? The worst thing, worse than the lost money, were the lies I told my husband over that period in time..

I stopped gambling, placing my last bet on November 6, 2020 I disclosed to my husband on the evening of November the 7th 2020. At the time of this writing, I have not gambled since.

To say he was furious would be minimizing what I did to him; the betrayal he felt after everything he had done for me in our marriage was unfathomable. At the time of this writing, we are slowly rebuilding our marriage. I know I have to earn back his trust and his respect; I pray I can earn his forgiveness too. Our marriage is strong, we have been together for 29 years, neither of us want to throw that away. I am getting help. I see a gambling addictions counsellor. I have blocked on-line casinos from my devices. I participate in online help for compulsive gamblers. I journal. I read self help books and books from gamblers anonymous. I have reached out to two of my brothers, Bob and Bill, and my sister-in law Mona, without their support I would not be where I am at today. I am terrified for Rob's family to hear of this news. If I haven't already told them they will read it here. I pray for their understanding and forgiveness, but I am aware that it may be too much to ask.

Upon disclosing my gambling problem to some of my family, I learned that I was not the only one with this disorder, I had other family members whom were also afflicted with problem gambling.

In reaching out for help, I learned from other compulsive gamblers that I was not alone, there are a lot of us, from many backgrounds and many financial positions, and that despite our differences we all have one similarity, we chased the losses and the casinos always won. We were good at lying and we lost way more than just money. We lost our self-respect, put our marriages and family relationships at risk, some lost their homes and entire savings and from what I learned, we all had gut wrenching guilt and shame. For me, I had never hated myself more. If you're in this position, please do not go through it alone, there is some really good help and support out there. You made a terrible mistake, but you are not a terrible person.

In "becoming" a compulsive gambler, I learned something about my mental health. I learned about my obsessive-compulsive behaviour. I truly understand how unwell I am. I try not to beat myself up, but I do every day, as I am barraged with guilt, shame and humiliation. I see the pain my husband is in. The pain that I have caused. Growing up with a narcissist, I am very good at wearing guilt, shame and humiliation. I am also very good at stuffing my own thoughts and feelings down. I learned how to from a very young age. It was how I coped.

I also learned from my counsellor about the likely link between my mental health and my gambling problem. It made sense how I sought out gambling to fulfill what was missing in my life. The excitement and adrenaline rush of gambling replaced the loss from my career and the void from other things in my life. Please understand that I am not excusing myself, I accept full responsibility for my choices.

I am new in my recovery, but I am determined to use my obsessive-compulsiveness for good, to help me get better. I have no urge to gamble. No desire. For me, I choose my marriage over gambling. I only pray I am not too late.

This journey has been a rough and sometimes rocky road. My husband and I remain committed to our marriage. I am open and transparent with him. I no longer have anything to hide and boy oh boy does that ever feel good! He is learning to trust me again.

CHAPTER 7

LOSS

On November 3, 2012 my step father, Bob Wilson, passed away, I held his hand as he took his last breath. He was 81 years old. His last words that were spoken to me the night before resonated; "I'm sorry to ditch out on you kid. I know that I'm now the second dad you've had to say good bye to." I was shattered.

On December 31, 2014 our family dog, Mia, passed away unexpectedly after suffering a fatal seizure. She was 11 years old and I must have cried for 48 hours straight. She was a pet, but she was a part of our family.

On January 7, 2015 my father-in-law, Don Hill, passed away of brain cancer. He was 83 years old. He was a kind and caring man and was well respected in our community. My husband and I were with him when he died in a palliative care home. This experience was so hard. It's hard to watch a person that you love die, even if they are elderly. I loved and respected him so very much.

In February 2016, my brother Bill's wife, Lorna, fell dramatically ill. It started with a stomach ache that went from a pain rated from 1 to a score of 10 within as many minutes. She would languish in hospital for days before being diagnosed with cancer. First though she went septic and then went into coma on the operating table. My brother nearly lost the love of his life then.

Ever so slowly we believed that she was recovering. She had many surgeries throughout the months that followed. She was on death's doorstep many times, but Lorna was a fighter and against the odds she pulled through and came out of her coma. The doctor's believed they got all the cancer from her. An oncologist however wanted her to have chemotherapy to ensure all the cancer was gone, "if it comes back" he said "she will not survive..." While Lorna was undergoing her first chemo treatment, Bill and I were texting one another when suddenly and without warning his text messages stopped. Later that day, I would learn that Lorna suffered a severe allergic reaction to the chemotherapy. Fortunately for Lorna, Bill was a paramedic and when she started convulsing in front of him, he knew what to do to help her. Lorna was then taken to hospital by ambulance where it was determined she suffered a severe allergic reaction to the chemo; anaphylactic shock. She was offered another chemotherapy concoction, one that was more costly and only available to patients that suffered a severe reaction, such as Lorna's. Before they could administer this, however, they had to wait for Lorna to recover from the effects of the horrendous allergic reaction.

In short, she developed what was thought to be a migraine headache that just wouldn't go away. Bill advocated for his wife and tests later revealed that not only had the cancer grown back, but it was everywhere in her body and in her head, behind her eyes and in her jaw; wherever the doctors looked and tested it showed more cancer. She was riddled with this horrendous disease and was given months to live.

She was 56 years old, her and Bill had been married for 25 years, they never had children and Bill would be left alone. Lorna asked me to take care of Bill. She was more worried about him than she was for herself. She had her faith and knew she would be taken care of in the afterlife. Despite her beliefs, or maybe because of them, she fought gallantly. Lorna was eventually placed in palliative care and on July 24, 2016 she succumbed to cancer with Bill at her side and me down the hall.

Five months! On February 13, 2016 Lorna said to Bill "I'm going to the gym for a workout" only to return minutes later with a pain in her stomach and within minutes after that was writhing in pain. It didn't make any sense; she was a healthy young woman.

She exercised, she didn't smoke, rarely drank and she practised self-care. She was an educated woman and was an articulate and caring therapist and animal advocate. Most importantly, she was without a doubt my brother's soul mate.

During this five-month journey to Hell, I spent a lot of time with Bill and Lorna. I tried to help and support Bill the best that I could. It was heart wrenching and gut wrenching all at the same time. During this timeframe my daughter and her husband would separate. I remember leaving Lorna's side and taking a phone call shortly thereafter, it was my son in law and he was suicidal. Fortunately, I was able to talk him down from committing suicide, and with him feeling better, I was able to return to my brother's side.

When my son in law talked about suicide, I remembering feeling like my heart was being ripped out of my chest, he had three children to think of – my grandchildren! I was in Vancouver and he was in Port Alberni; a 90-minute ferry trip and a 3 hour drive away.

What do I do? How do I help him? I cannot leave my brother and yet how do I stay? Emotionally I was a mess yet I felt that I had to stay strong and keep myself together for everyone. I certainly couldn't tell Bill or Lorna; they were already dealing with too much. I explained to my son in law where I was and why, I recall saying to him if he doesn't get help immediately that I was phoning the police to come and help him. Together we agreed on an action plan and he assured me he wouldn't harm himself. He was able to stay true to his word. Thank you again God.

During this time, I would travel back and forth from Port Alberni to Vancouver. On one of my stays at home I developed pain in my lower abdomen. I was able to see my gynaecologist and he immediately did a biopsy. It was painful, but I chose to do it in his office and without anaesthetic because I was scared and wanted the results as quickly as possible. It was because of all of my symptoms; he was concerned that it was cancer. Within a few days my test results would come back as benign. Thank you yet again, God!

After Lorna's death, I watched my brother go from a strong independent man to a shell of his former self. He is slowly now moving forward from this tragic loss, but it has been a very long journey.

Bill and I have been through a lot together and this was no exception. Lorna's death impacted me wholeheartedly. I miss her and our conversations. If anything virtuous came from Lorna's dying, it is that I reconnected with her mother and became friends with her sister, brother and their families.

The long journey and the eventual death of Lorna impacted me greatly. My heart hurt for my brother. My heart hurt for Lorna. I will never forget the shock on her face when she learned that she had been handed a death sentence. Lorna and I talked in private. In truth, mostly she talked and I cried openly. She said she wanted Bill to live life after she was gone. "I want him to laugh and I want him to fall in love again. He's got to go on living…" I thanked her then, for being Bill's wife, his partner in the truest sense of the word. I thanked her for getting him up to dance at my wedding. (Bill did not like to dance.) We laughed and we cried together.

I remember being at her funeral and I looked over at my brother. There was a line-up of well-wishers waiting to talk to him. I could see that he had no more to give. I took him by the hand and said "I'm taking you out of here for a while." He responded "take me, hold me, don't ever let me go." Once again, my heart shattered.

Then on October 22, 2018 my niece, my brother Bob's daughter, passed away. She was 46 years old and died as a result of complications from a car accident that occurred where she was living in Saudi Arabia. Her death was heart shattering. She was a beautiful and educated young woman. Our family is not the same without her and she is sorely missed. Tanya, my forever princess.

CHAPTER 8

RECOVERY AND HOPE

I met with my psychiatrist three weeks after my last gambling bet. In a nutshell, he explained to me that had I had told him earlier about my gambling (such as before it became a problem) he would have increased some of my medication, and my therapy, then perhaps I wouldn't be in the situation I'm in now. He further explained that because of my anxiety, combined with my compulsiveness, and the Covid-19 isolation (boredom, loneliness etc.,) I reached out to a (negative) source to fill my void. He encouraged me to keep with counselling and stay on my medications.

To date, I am in counselling, see my psychiatrist regularly, participate weekly in online compulsive gamblers meetings, journal, meditate, exercise and read a lot of books around recovery including Gambler's Anonymous, as well as, reading for enjoyment. I participate in an online workshop for problem gamblers. I am part of a book club and when COVID allows, our small group of women meets monthly in person, otherwise we meet online via zoom. Most importantly I keep in regular contact with, and I am honest with, all of my supports, but most important of all, this keeps me honest with myself and with my husband. As a result, my marriage is becoming stronger again. Our love is true and we have hope for a future together.

I am not inferring that all is easy and perfect in my marriage, because it's not. It's an emotional rollercoaster; we both have some really great days and we have some days where we are angry and don't like each other very much. For a woman with my history of abuse it's very easy to feel victimized, while at the same time, it's very easy for my husband to be punitive. He is still raw and hurting. I am new in my recovery and plus I have a whole gambit of other issues. This alone makes for a rocky road. We do love each other, a lot. However, he has lost respect and trust in me and without that how does one rebuild a marriage? I am told by other compulsive gamblers to be open and transparent and accountable for my mistake and I am. I will not however continue to beat myself up for my horrible transgression. I did a horrible thing, but I am not a horrible person. Continuously berating myself is not going to help anyone, least of all me in my recovery. In actuality, I have learned through the professionals, that continuously beating myself up is a risk factor to start gambling again.

I continue to take all my medications as prescribed. I keep myself busy every day. I use a software blocker so that I cannot access any online sites even if I wanted to. I am responsible for my choices. I have hope.

I continue to work on my mental health. It's really challenging to advocate for myself and my heart goes out to those who try to do it alone. I am fortunate, I have my rock; my husband. I also have my children. I especially have Bill, Bob and Mona. I believe that having a support system in place is a fundamental part in personal growth, healing and recovery. In short, don't try and go it alone.

I am hopeful to be able to return to some type of work even if it should be volunteer work. When I'm well, I would like to be able to help others, who like me, struggle to become the person that I was before, <u>except</u> I want to be stronger and healthier. I want to be a person that practises self-care not just promotes or preaches it! That is my life goal and it is what keeps me moving forward each day. Recovery and hope for a better me.

For me self-care means being kind and forgiving of myself, taking time to see and feel life, to meditate, exercise, eat well, journal, have a social life, spend time with my husband, our children and grandchildren, but most importantly it is about being aware of myself and my surroundings. It's also about reaching out to others; my therapist, my group meetings. I love to sing and dance, and as I have learned from my brother Bill, it is to be present in the physical and spiritual world.

Life is amazing, all we have to do is embrace it. Shifting our attitudes changes life's outcome, because it changes our thoughts and beliefs.

.. and remember, wherever you are at in your personal journey, you are not alone.

Reach out, the help is there.

I stated earlier that I want to be "stronger" and healthier and when I say that I am implying that because I am unwell, I am "weak." For me, this is one of my greatest hurdles; the opposite of strong is weak and sadly that is how I view myself, not others, just myself. I view those that reach out for help as demonstrating a strength, yet for me I see and judge myself as weak. All I can say is that I am working on myself and through intensive therapy I hope to come out the other side and like my therapist says, instead of viewing myself as weak, why not understand myself as human. She's right of course. I do have distorted thinking and that is something that, although it is ingrained in me, I can counter these distorted thoughts with a healthier attitude. Instead of telling myself "I am weak" I can simply say "I am human."

I have hope for a better me. I got a tattoo on the inside of my right arm with a turtle and a butterfly along with the words "it's my turn" signifying that it's my turn to take care of me, whereas the turtle signifies a slow and steady pace forward and the butterfly signifies new life.

I pray that this book may help others that have been in similar situations to know that they are not alone and that we always have hope. I also pray that this may help others to be more understanding and empathetic towards those that have experienced and lived through domestic violence, sexual abuse and addictions.

Domestic violence is in and of itself difficult for others to understand why a person would stay in an abusive relationship. There are many reasons; lack of support, nowhere to go, financial reasons and fear are just some of the rationale that many victims grapple with. For me, the fear of failure, of being killed by my abuser and fear of how I may be judged by others were huge factors for me. However, when my abusers had illicit affairs, I accepted that as a behaviour that other people would not unjustly judge me for, but would instead be more understanding and compassionate about why I left the relationships. That is, it would be socially acceptable for me to leave my husband because he had an affair as opposed to undergoing abuse. Unfairly, there is still so much blame and politic around the victims of domestic violence.

Sexual abuse of a child is, more often than not, normally something that people don't blame the victim for. It is in this incidence where people hold the offender more accountable. Sadly, for the child, the victim usually blames themselves. I know that I did and sometimes still do.

Growing up with a narcissist parent was the most challenging and biggest struggle of my life that continues to traumatize and haunt me to this day. I continue to battle my childhood demons and the scars that my mother inflicted upon me. In part I believe this is because she is still alive and I choose to continue to have her in my life. I think that the biggest challenge for me is that I always worry about being judged by others. Whether it is a perfect stranger, a colleague, a close friend or a family member. If and when I am judged in a negative fashion, I take it exceptionally personally and almost always blame myself despite the reason for the judgement or the source. I have a very difficult time forgiving myself when I make even the slightest mistake and I carry that feeling with me for many years. For example, about five years ago I pulled out into traffic when I didn't have the right away. Two women laid on their horns, stopped and while glaring at me shook their heads. I mouthed I'm sorry, but it didn't matter they continued to glare at me. I burst into tears and to this day I feel as though that incident just happened. My throat tightens and I feel nauseous because of what I did. Deep down I know this isn't normal, but I cannot shake the feeling. Guilt and shame are two ingrained traits that a narcissist parent inflicts upon their children.

Addictive behaviour is difficult and challenging to understand, the professionals say that there is actually a change in the brain's chemistry. Is addiction a disease or a choice? Personally, I feel that for myself I initially chose to gamble, but something happened to me that got out of control. It wasn't that I didn't care or that I made a conscious decision to blow through money I didn't have, I was out of control. I no longer had control over my behaviour. Then something happened that caused me to stop before completely running out of money. I don't know what that was, but for me, I had gone too far. I thank my God, my higher power, for helping me before it was too late.

I think that because I experienced so much abuse both as a child and young adult, that it has also somehow shaped me to be a better me. That is, I believe I am more compassionate of victims, witnesses and offenders. I believe I am a compassionate and caring mom. I always wanted my children to know that no matter what their experiences, beliefs or actions; they would ALWAYS have me to turn to. My parental love is unconditional and that I will always, always, go to bat for them, whether or not they are right or wrong or somewhere in between. I never ever want my children to feel that they have nowhere to go or no one to turn to.

AUTHORS NOTE

This memoir was very difficult for me to write. My training and background as a probation officer includes writing reports for the court. In those reports they had to be factual and without emotion, a memoir, on the other hand, is to include emotion. I hope that I encapsulated emotion here. In addition, I further struggled because I don't want to hurt any of the people I wrote about and whom are significant people in my life. Some parts of my memoir include their stories and it's such a delicate balance to tell my own story without betraying the experiences of anyone else. If I did that, I am sorry, the memories I spoke of are mine and mine alone.

At one of the readings of this manuscript, my husband said that I was not sharing enough and that I needed to go into more detail. My brother Bill also read my manuscript, he felt the same way and also said he felt that I was trying to protect each of the people that I wrote about. I went back and edited as per their suggestions. I hope I did them justice.

I also struggled with my writing, because one of my coping mechanisms included "blocking" certain painful memories. My therapist then taught me about compartmentalizing, (when a person suppresses their thoughts and emotions) she suggested I have a box, or a compartment, where I could put notes to myself about things I was suppressing while writing my memoir. I did this. I purchased a floral box with butterflies on the outside and as I wrote I placed little notes to myself that were too painful to write about or were too painful to expand upon. When I am ready, I am hopeful that her and I will delve into those during our therapy sessions.

Thank you for reading my very first book! I would love to hear from you. Please email me at darlene0511@icloud.com

Or check out my webpage @ www.darleneahill.ca

Warmly,
Darlene Hill

It is with a heavy heart that I write that just prior to my final edits on this book that my youngest daughter Elisabeth's life partner, Philip, passed away suddenly and accidentally on March 27, 2021 Another great and tragic loss.

ACKNOWLEDGEMENTS

A Woman's Story, never would have happened the way it did without the loving support of my family; especially true of my husband Rob, my brothers Bill and Bob and my sister-in law Mona as well as counsellors, therapists and doctors. I thank each of my children because without their support I never would have made it this far. Thank you, Christine, Lisa and Elisabeth. Thank-you Kimmy. I love you all.

I would also like to thank "My Team" at Tellwell Publishing, without each of you my book would not have been possible! Thank you to my project consultant Jennifer Chapin, with special thanks to my Project Manager Charlyne Calisang, Jessica Kirby (editor), Nikolai (book cover designer), Michael John Paul Lapar (book interior designer) and Angela Gascon (marketing consultant and web designer). Yay, we did it!!!

LIST OF HELPFUL RESOURCES

- Gamblers Anonymous
- www.gamtalk.org
- B.C. Problem Gambling Helpline 1-888-795-6111 (24 hrs)
- Gamblers National Helpline 1-800-522-4700
- Assaulted Women's Helpline 1-866-863-0511 (24 hrs)
- www.bcresponsiblegambling.ca
- www.problemgambling.ca

www.ingramcontent.com/pod-product-compliance
Lightning Source LLC
LaVergne TN
LVHW041540060526
838200LV00037B/1073